FIGHTING THE VIRUS

HOW TO BOOST YOUR BODY'S IMMUNE RESPONSE AND FIGHT VIRUSES AND BACTERIA NATURALLY

JOSEPH VEEBE

Other Books in this Series:

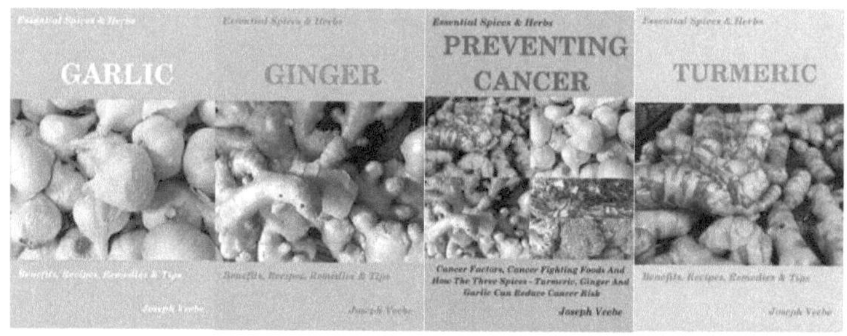

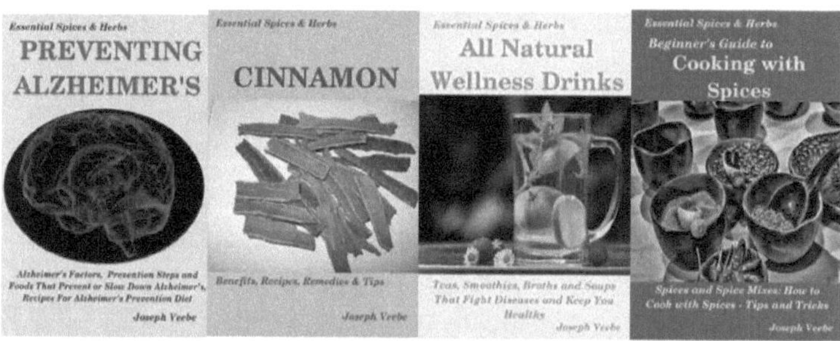

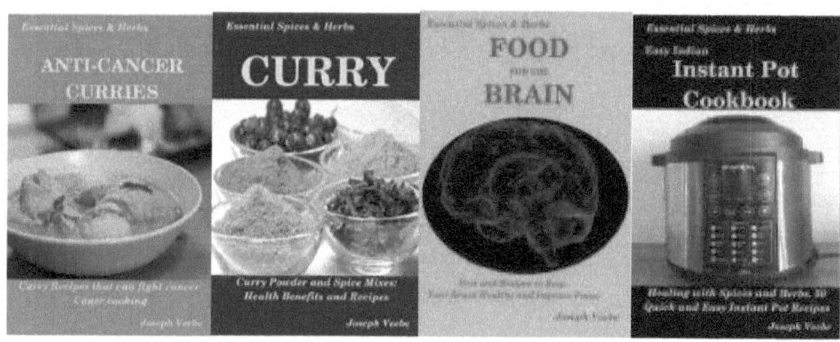

TABLE OF CONTENTS

CHAPTER 1. INTRODUCTION

INTRODUCTION

This book is a result of my research into natural ways of dealing with infectious diseases as a supplemental and/or alternative treatment to modern medicine and clinical practices. While modern medicine has advanced leaps and bounds over the last several decades in treating many diseases, our modern lifestyle has also caused new health conditions and new diseases that were not known in the years past.

Ancient tribes used many natural substances as part of medical practices based on their evidence-based effectiveness against particular conditions. Some of these natural substances (herbs, spices, and others) have been undergoing scientific studies to validate these age-old claims. While some of these claims have been proven to be of substance and others not so much, it clear that these natural methods hold value as a potentially safe alternative or complement to chemical drugs that are often costly and comes with many side effects.

A healthy lifestyle is critical for a healthy body that can fight many diseases. A healthy lifestyle typically improves the body's immune system making it difficult for external particles (viruses) and bacteria to infiltrate or once infiltrated to thrive and cause damage.

ANTIBIOTICS AND ANTIVIRALS

Modern medicines such as antibiotics and antiviral vaccines have revolutionized treatment options for humans. The use of antibiotics and antiviral vaccines has saved countless millions of people in the last 80-100 years since the invention of antiseptic (Lysozyme) and Penicillin by Alexander Fleming. Over the next several decades, vaccines targeted for various virus strains were invented further progressing the treatment options for many infectious diseases.

Indiscriminate use of antibiotics has also created another set of problems:

- Bacteria have become more adaptive and resistant to standard treatments. In some cases, normal antibiotics have become ineffective or need much larger doses to be effective.
- While antibiotics do kill the harmful bacteria and help you recover quickly, it has side effects in that it can also kill the friendly bacteria in your digestive tract impacting your gut health which can cause diarrhea, heartburn, constipation, and a general reduction in the body's immunity.

While for severe conditions, antibiotics are probably the only option, antibiotics need to be administered carefully so that the above two problems are minimized.

The story of antiviral vaccines is no different than that of antibiotics. While vaccines are effective to the exact strain of the virus, it becomes ineffective for a different strain as the virus mutates. For a new virus mutation, we will need to find a new vaccine to be effective. These new viruses could result in major outbreaks or pandemics depending how fast they spread and how soon a treatment or vaccine could be invented. Given how people around the world are closely connected, any such new virus outbreak to spread indiscriminately before any effective treatment options devised to treat or slow down such outbreaks. The recent pandemic due to coronavirus is a classic example where viruses are spreading indiscriminately in a globalized world with no effective treatment options immediately available to date.

SOME OF THE MAJOR PANDEMICS TO HIT HUMANKIND

The following is a history of some of the major bacterial/viral outbreaks that caused pandemics and resulted in large scale deaths until either a treatment/vaccine was found, or population developed immunity to the virus.

- Black Death or Bubonic Plague (1346-1353)
    - Death toll: 75-200 million
    - Cause: Bacterium *Yersinia Pestis*
    - Where: Europe, Africa, and Asia
    - End – through quarantines and improved personal hygiene
- Cholera – multiple pandemics
    - Death toll: 2M+ over 7 distinct outbreaks at various times spanning 19th and 20th century
    - Cause bacterium *Vibrio cholera*
    - End – through vaccination

- Influenza pandemic (1918)
  - Death toll: 20-50 million
  - Cause: Influenza virus Type A, B or C
  - Where: All over the globe
  - End – Influenza vaccine
- HIV/AIDS pandemic (1981-2015+)
  - Death toll: 36 million
  - Cause: HIV/AIDS
  - Where: Africa and the rest of the world
  - End – HIV/AIDS continues but manageable with new treatments
- Coronavirus (2019-2020)
  - Death toll: Not determined
  - Cause: coronavirus
  - Where: all over the world
  - End – TBD

Besides these, there are other pandemics such as Asian flu (death toll 2M), Influenza, and other flu pandemics.

Coronavirus is an ongoing pandemic at the time of writing this book. Coronavirus has caused major havoc in the lives of people all around the world driving almost two-thirds of the world population (5 billion people) to quarantine and social isolation. In addition, financial markets have been battered to the levels not seen since the great depression driving the world to the brink of a major recession.

Quarantine and confinement have caused major hardships to a lot of people, especially the working class who are unable to get out of the home to make their livelihood. In many third world countries, the situation is even more acute. Industries such as restaurants, bars, hotels, transportation, and aviation have been hit hard.

The impact of coronavirus has been unprecedented and complicated due to several factors such as global economic integration, increased mobility and travel, high levels of population, the difference in cultures and ideologies, and high interdependency between people and countries around the world.

At the time of writing this book, there are over a million confirmed cases around the world and possibly 5 times that number of cases exist but not tested. There are more than 80,000 people identified as dead due to the virus with the death toll possibly rising as the pandemic is expected to peak in the near future.

The reason for including the above information is to show that how much ever advanced our science and medicine are today, pandemics are real, and such large scale viral or bacterial infections can have devastating consequences in today's globalized world with over 7 billion population with several large cities that are overcrowded.

Fortunately for us, lessons from history, public and population health advancements, medical and scientific advancements, and data science prepare us to respond to such mass scale infections with a coordinated effort from around the world. In addition, we have the luxury of multiple teams and best minds across the world working on a solution in parallel while quarantine efforts are put in place to contain the transmission.

WHAT THIS BOOK IS ABOUT

What can we do as individuals to improve our health and immunity so that we are less prone to get an infection and fight it vigorously in case of getting one?

The answer lies in lifestyle changes that improve immunity and keep our body in optimum health naturally to have a fair chance to fight these infections as medications or vaccines for a new virus or bacteria is yet to be invented.

This book is an effort to compile such natural substances that can improve immunity and can fight viral and bacterial infections. The book also gives you some ideas and recipes about cooking up some nature-based remedies at home along with food preparations that contain ingredients to fight infections.

Chapter 2. Human Immune System

The immune system is the human body's multi-layer defense mechanism to keep the human body healthy from disease-causing organisms, malfunctioning human body cells, and external particles or substances.

The first line of defense - Skin

The skin forms a shield against any harmful organism or particle that it comes in contact with. The outer layer of the skin not only forms a protective layer for internal organs but also secrets chemicals that kill potential invaders. The epidermis or outer skin sheds 30-40 thousand dead cells a day in its effort to fight these invaders. Keeping your skin healthy is important, therefore, in your fight against these external invaders.

The first line of defense – Mucus and Cilia

The air we breathe contains foreign particles and bacteria. As we breathe in, these particles and bacteria come in contact with **mucus** throughout the respiratory system and get stuck. **Cilia** are hair-like structures that protrude from the cell body and they sweep the mucus into the throat for coughing it out for swallowing. This action helps prevent harmful external particles and bacteria from entering into human cells and harming them.

In case you wonder if the swallowed mucus infected with bacteria is harmful, the answer is it is generally not as the stomach acid works to neutralize them.

THE FIRST LINE OF DEFENSE – SALIVA

Maybe you don't do this as a grown-up but when you were a kid, what is the first thing you do when you cut your finger? Your answer, most likely, is putting the finger in the mouth. It is because saliva contains antibacterial compounds besides digestive enzymes that can break down or kill many kinds of bacteria. There are, however, many other kinds of bacteria that can survive saliva.

THE FIRST LINE OF DEFENSE – STOMACH ACID

Stomach acid not only breaks down your food but also kills any bacteria swallowed through mucus or entered the digestive system as part of the food.

THE SECOND LINE OF DEFENSE – WHITE BLOOD CELLS

If the external invaders are able to penetrate the first line of defense and get inside the body, for example, through a cut on your skin, then white blood cells start fighting the invaders.

White blood cells are usually circulated through the blood to all parts of the body and remain in the bloodstream. However, if invaders are detected within the cell body, the white blood cells enter the body cells to fight off and neutralize the invader.

Body cells contain a number of structures called organelles, these organelles such as mitochondrion, the chloroplast, and the lysosome, etc. are like organs in the cell body and have specific functions.

Virus, once they enter the body cells, take over the various organelles and convert them into "virus making factories" resulting in a swollen cell containing thousands of viruses. These swollen cells eventually burst to spread thousands of viruses to adjacent body cells.

Some of the white blood cells are known as phagocytes which can detect foreign invaders and engulf them so that these harmful particles/viruses or bacteria are neutralized preventing them from harming body cells.

THE SECOND LINE OF DEFENSE – INTERFERON

Interferon is a protein released by body cells usually as a response to virus infection. Interferon has the property of inhibiting virus replication and virus' ability to attack other cells

What happens to already infected cells? This is where T-Cells come in. T-Cells are often called "natural killer" cells that have the ability to detect and selectively attack those infected cells and kill them. T-Cells will continue to do this "search and destroy" operation until no more infected cells are found.

THE SECOND LINE OF DEFENSE – INFLAMMATION

Inflammatory response by injured or infected body cells is a mechanism by which it raises the alarm signals for the attention of the body's defensive mechanisms. Injured body cells release histamine, a chemical substance that helps with the inflammatory response, during which:

- Capillaries dilate and swelling happens
- Pyrogens are released which reaches hypothalamus and body temperature rises
- Pain receptors are activated
- All these actions result in white blood cells to flock to the affected area

TWO DIVISIONS OF THE IMMUNE SYSTEM

- Cell-mediated
- Antibody-mediated

The cell-mediated immune system is centered around how white blood cells – phagocytes and T-cells fight harmful invaders. While phagocytes eat or swallow invaders and neutralize them, T-cells directly attacks and kill them.

The antibody-mediated immune system is controlled by antibodies and forms the third line of defense in the body's immune system

THIRD LINE OF DEFENSE – ANTIBODIES

The human body's layered defense mechanisms ensure that most of the harmful invaders are neutralized at the first or second line of defense. If by any chance, these viruses and bacteria were able to penetrate the first two layers of defense and infect the body, this triggers the third line of defense – production of antibodies

- Antibodies are proteins that latch on to foreign particles and damage or slow them down
- Each antibody binds to one specific antigen

Antibodies are produced by B-cells component on white blood cells in collaboration with both phagocytes and T-cells. The antibodies targeted for the specific type of foreign particles so that they can latch on to it.

IMMUNITY AND ILLNESS

When an external invader (or particle) penetrated the first two lines of defense and entered into the body and started affecting body cells, the person falls sick and remains ill until the 3rd line of defense kicks in. If the external invader or particle was already known to body and quickly recognized, antibodies are crafted right away, and these are particles are neutralized even before the person falls sick. This person is considered immune to this kind of external invaders.

Immunity is thus defined as the resistance of the human body to a disease-causing organism or a harmful substance. Immunity can be classified into two types

- Active Immunity
- Passive Immunity

The simple difference between active immunity and passive immunity is that, in the case of active immunity, the individual body produces antibodies and in the case passive, the antibodies have been passed on to you from your mother.

In most cases, active immunity is attained through the exposure of the body to antigen, either inadvertently or on purpose.

Inadvertent exposure results in the body falling sick due to the actual disease-causing antigen. Your body fought and won the disease by creating antibodies. Now the body remembers these antigens and is prepared for it, should they enter the body again.

Planned exposure, is through vaccination, where the body is exposed to an antigen that is killed or weakened. Your body detects and fights them by creating antibodies. Now the body knows about this antigen and is prepared for it.

Through planned exposure or vaccination, several diseases that used to be prevalent in the middle ages, such as polio and smallpox have been eradicated completely.

Some of these vaccines, such as for smallpox, last a lifetime while others such as for flu need annual or periodic vaccinations as these viruses mutate to new forms that the body cannot recognize anymore.

While the planned immunity through vaccines is essential and is prescribed in mostly all countries against the various epidemics that happened in the past (measles, cholera, etc.), our body is left to fend itself against any new or novel pathogens until a vaccine or medicine is invented.

The best way to defend these yet to appear pathogens is by keeping your body ready to fight by improving the body's immunity and viral fighting capabilities through natural medicines and lifestyle adjustments.

IMMUNE DISORDERS

Allergies

Allergies are the body's response to foreign particles that the body recognizes incorrectly as harmful and go on a war against them. In many cases, these are harmless substances such as pollen, eggs, peanuts, and many others.

As part of the response, the immune system releases antibodies as a message to cells to stop these substances. The cells produce histamine which causes blood vessels to expand and generate other allergy symptoms.

In some people, the immune system reacts to these harmless substances by launching an immune response which causes sneezing, coughing, runny nose, and watery eyes. In some cases, allergic reactions may be much severe and can cause shortness of breath, wheezing, chest congestion, skin rashes, and hives. Serious cases of an allergic reaction can lead to anaphylaxis where breathing becomes really hard, tightening of the throat, nausea or vomiting and fainting, and dizziness. These conditions will require immediate treatment.

Anti-histamines block the effect of histamine and provide allergy relief.

Acquired Immune Deficiency Syndrome (AIDS)

AIDS was discovered in 1983 and is caused by the Human Immunodeficiency Virus (HIV). These viruses specifically target T-cells and since normal body cells are not affected immune response is not launched by the body.

The HIV virus does not really kill you. BUT these viruses shut down the immune system and as a result, even common diseases such as flu or common cold which were easily defeated by your immune system now become serious and could be life-threatening.

Once acquired, the HIV virus could remain dormant and no effects for months or for even years.

AIDS is transmitted by external contacts like blood transfusions or contaminated needles, etc.

Autoimmune diseases

When the immune system attacks own healthy body cells instead of invading foreign matter, the condition is called an autoimmune disease. There are eighty or so known autoimmune conditions affecting about 24million people in the united states. Some common autoimmune diseases are listed below:

Lupus: Lupus is a condition where the body's immune system attacks healthy cells in many parts of the body including the skin, joints, kidney, heart, brain, lungs, etc. causing inflammation and damage. It affects about 1.5 million people in the US

Rheumatoid Arthritis: Immune system attacks joints causing inflammation, swelling, and pain resulting in long term joint damage if left untreated. It affects about 1.5 million people in the US.

Type 1 diabetes: Immune system targets insulin creating cells in the pancreas and causes damage or destroys them. Since these cells cannot make enough insulin (which regulates blood sugar), blood sugar levels elevate to dangerous levels. Type 1 diabetes is usually diagnosed in childhood and affects about 1.25 million Americans.

Multiple Sclerosis: The immune system attacks myelin which acts as a protective sheath for nerves around the spinal cord, brain, and optic nerves. The impact could be slowness in movement, slurry speech, dizziness, loss of vision, and general weakness. MS could be genetic, and women are more susceptible than men.

Inflammatory Bowel Disease (IBD): Impacting more than 3 million people in the US, IBD can cause severe diarrhea and abdominal pain due to inflammation in the digestive tract. Ulcerative colitis and Chron's disease fall under IBD and are chronic.

Psoriasis: The immune system attacks healthy skin cells causing redness, itching, and scaling of the skin. It affects more than 8 million people in the US. Psoriasis can result in systemic inflammation impacting vital organs such as the heart.

Other autoimmune diseases include **vasculitis** (swelling and inflammation of blood vessels), **thyroid disease** where the production of thyroid hormones is impacted (overproduction – Graves' disease; underproduction - Hashimoto thyroiditis), **scleroderma** (skin) and many others which are less common.

While it is not scientifically proven nor FDA approved, some of the natural substances we discussed earlier have shown to help improve general immunity and prevent or slow down some of the immune conditions discussed above.

Chapter 3. General Strategies for Boosting Immunity

A Good Night's Sleep

The whole body uses sleep as a restorative process to recover from all the work the body did during waking hours. New research has shown that lack of sleep can increase the risk of many diseases and the body's readiness to fight diseases. Some studies have shown the need for proper (REM stage) sleep for flushing out toxins from the brain. The body uses sleep time to re-distribute T-cells to lymph nodes and other parts of the body. Studies have found that sleep deprived-body is more susceptible to a virus than a well-rested body.

Tips for sound sleep:

- Establish a regular schedule for sleep. A regular sleep cycle reinforces the body's natural clock and helps you to have a better sleep.
- Establish a routine and mood. A glass of warm milk, a hot bath, stretching, diary or journal entries, or dim lights may help.
- Switch off electronics – phones, laptops, TVs, etc. are huge distractions and impediments to sound sleep.
- Relax. If you are stressed it is hard to sleep. Use one of the relaxation techniques to decompress before sleep.
- Snoring or sleep apnea. Get tested and treated. It can make a huge difference in sleep quality.

DIET

Diet is one of the most important factors in keeping a healthy body. Eating properly and avoid unhealthy eating is a major factor in weight control, building immunity, avoiding autoimmune diseases (to an extent) and also speedy recovery if you develop a health condition.

Here are some recommendations on healthy eating:

- Avoid foods that cause inflammation such as sugars and refined carbs (white rice, white/bleached flour, pasta).
- Include anti-inflammatory foods (including spices and herbs) into the diet.
- Eat a lot of fish. Omega-3 fats containing DHA help prevent Alzheimer's and dementia by countering plaque formation. Include oily fishes like salmon, tuna, sardines, mackerel, trout, etc. in your diet.
- Eat a lot of fruits and vegetables, especially colorful vegetables.
- Include the Mediterranean diet as part of your diet regiment.
- Practice the DASH diet.
- Eat whole foods and grains.
- Drink more tea.
- Eat more nuts and seeds.

- Avoid fast foods, fried foods, and packaged foods.
- Avoid processed foods.
- Eat foods that strengthen your digestive system and consequently improve your immunity.
- Eat fresh meals.
- Cook at home.

STRESS MANAGEMENT

Our bodies respond to stress in many different ways. From an immunity standpoint, acute stress or chronic stress condition compromises the body's response in a negative way. Stress can inhibit digestion of the food you eat. This can impact the health of the digestive system and may result in ulcers. Major stress or depression can cause a measurable decrease in the number of T-Cells or a type of white cell that is key in defending against viruses and bacteria.

A weakened immune system due to stress is susceptible to a number of diseases including viral and bacterial infections.

Below are some techniques for stress management:

Breathing

Breathing is one of the "in the moment" stress management techniques.

- Deep breathing. Take a number of deep breaths. With each deep breath, the body relaxes progressively.
- Abdominal breathing. Place hands on belly. Hands should go out with your belly on the inhale, in on the exhale. Repeat until feeling relaxed.
- Breath counting. 5 seconds of inhaling followed by 5 seconds of exhaling. Also, you can hold your breath for 5 seconds before exhaling.

Channel your inner peace

- Practice regular meditation.
- Practice daily prayer.
- Regular religious practice. Attending church service, going to temple, synagogue, or mosque.

Schedule daily **relaxation and mindfulness** exercises

- Practice yoga or tai chi.

Exercise helps reduce stress

- Pick up a game or a regular activity
- Try exercising or gym activities.
- Take up swimming.
- Try routinely running or walking.

Take time out for vacation

- All work and no play increases stress levels. Take time out. Schedule vacation time with friends or family.

Sense of humor/ laughing out loud

- Watch comedy films or shows.
- Try joking with friends and family.
- Or just laugh out loud for no reason.

Adopt a pet

- Pets help reduce stress.
- They also provide companionship.

REGULAR EXERCISE & PHYSICAL ACTIVITY

Being physically active and doing exercise has many health benefits and helps fight many diseases. From an immune system standpoint, exercise provides the following benefits:

- Body temperature rises as a result of physical exercise which helps slow down or prevent bacteria growth in the body and assists the body to fight the infection better. This function is similar to body raising the temperature by causing fever to help fight bacteria
- Exercise reduces stress. As we saw from the previous section, stress adversely impacts the immune system and lowers the count of T-cells.

- Physical activity may help flush out bacteria from the lungs due to improved breathing. This helps to reduce the possibility of viral or bacterial infections such as flu, cold, sore throat, etc.
- As blood circulation gets better with exercise, the antibodies and white blood cells (T-cells) can move around the body and fight infections rapidly improving the body's defense.

One does not need to spend hours in the gym every day to get benefits but 30 minutes a day will do the job. It is important, though, to come up with an exercise plan and stick to it every day. The ideal plan includes both cardio exercise and strength training. Besides these, a good beginner plan will include walking or swimming for 30 minutes or more a day.

For those people with a lot of time on their hands, especially after retirement, picking up a physical activity such as senior league for sports or even gardening can help. The key is to do these activities regularly.

Besides these, strength/resistance and weight training help you maintain not only your muscles but brain health as well. Add 2-3 weight sessions of 20-30 minutes into your weekly routine.

Another physical activity is to take up yoga or tai chi. Both of these not only help with strengthening your body and improving flexibility but sharpen your mind, improve concentration, and reduce stress.

It is never too late to start an exercise regimen and even small things count. The key is to get you on your feet. Doing household chores such as vacuuming and doing dishes also counts. Even when you need to work at a desk or watch TV, standing up to work or watch TV will be more beneficial than sitting for a majority of the time.

SMOKING, TOBACCO, DRUGS AND ALCOHOL

Smoking, the use of drugs, or excessive consumption of alcohol can have a negative impact on one's immunity besides causing other health conditions. The impact of smoking, drug use, and alcohol on overall health is well documented.

While pre-existing conditions play a part and maybe other hormonal and gender factors, one thing stands out is men by far outnumber women in smoking, drug, or alcohol use.

Some of the recent data relating to infectious disease show that the incidence rate, as well as the mortality rate for these infections, are higher in men than women. The data also shows that men outnumber women in the use of cigarettes, tobacco, drug, and alcohol use.

Making a lifestyle change of quitting smoking and drug use will have a significant impact on overall wellbeing and improving the body's natural immunity significantly.

MENTAL AND EMOTIONAL WELLBEING

In the previous sections, we focused on the physical aspects of wellbeing and lifestyle that have a positive effect on the immune system. A positive attitude and emotions can boost the body's immune system.

A study conducted at Pennsylvania University concluded that negative moods may change how the body's immune system reacts to potential threats and also that negative moods increased the risk of exacerbated inflammation.

Emotional wellbeing becomes even more important during a pandemic situation where people become isolated and are locked in their homes which can trigger depression, emotional distress (due to both physical and economic reasons), and boredom. Some suggestions to cope with such situation include:

Exercise: Find an exercise you like and make it a point to do it regularly. If you locked in, identify an exercise you can do indoors and stick to a schedule

Social connections: Social interaction helps to elevate your mood, reduce depression, etc. In the event, you are locked in, find ways to spend quality family time. Online collaboration and games are another way to stay connected while locked in.

Stress Reduction and Relaxation: Follow some of the techniques mentioned earlier. This helps improve emotional wellbeing.

As we discussed above, there are many lifestyles changes you can make that will improve your body's immune response. It is also clear that the older population, people who are sedentary, people who smoke or drink too much alcohol are more likely to a catch virus and more likely to have severe complications as a result. This is clearly evident in the recent pandemic at the time of this writing. It is all the more important, therefore, to take care of your body and prepare it for such outbreaks if you are 50 years or older.

CHAPTER 4. NATURAL WAYS OF FIGHTING VIRUS AND BACTERIA

This chapter will focus on ways to fight viruses and bacteria from infecting you and making your sick. There are clearly three aspects of this fight.

- Prevent coming in contact with bacteria in the first place.
- Improve the body's immunity by lifestyle changes so in case you come in contact with germs, the body is prepared to handle them. This strategy is discussed in detail in **Chapter 3.**
- Improve the body's defense and ability to fight bacteria and viruses through food and diet and incorporating natural substances in your everyday diet. This is discussed more in **Chapter 5.**

AVOIDING VIRUS AND BACTERIA

Personal hygiene

Personal hygiene plays a big part in avoiding germs and bacteria. Personal hygiene includes but not limited to the following:

- Toilet hygiene: Wash your hands with soap and water every time you go to the toilet
- Shower/Bath: Shower helps wash off any germs, dead skin cells, oils, etc. from your body and keep

your skin which is the first line of defense against germs clean.

- Teeth: dental hygiene helps fight cavities and gum disease which can cause other health conditions
- Nails: Germs can accumulate underneath nails
- Sickness hygiene: If you are sick, especially due to germs that are infectious, staying away from others, covering your mouth/nose while sneezing, cleaning any shared surfaces is important in not transmitting your disease to other people.

Washing hands

Typically, our hands touch many surfaces during the course a day. Germs on your hand can easily get inside your body through mouth, nose, ears, or eyes.

While washing hands is part of personal hygiene, it is important to highlight the importance of washing hands especially during flu season or in the middle of any contagious outbreaks. Essentially you want to make it to practice wash hands every time you go to the toilet, every time you touch an unclean surface or every time you touch public or shared things such as park benches, shopping carts, etc. It is recommended that you wash hands using soap and water for about 20 seconds. Both sides of the hand, wrist, between fingers, under the nails all needs to be thoroughly washed.

Using disinfectants to clean surfaces

Use disinfecting wipes, foam, or lotion such as Lysol, Clorox, Purell or others to wipe surfaces clean. Shopping carts, park benches, restaurant tables, door handles, airport, bus station, train station chairs, and seats on airplanes, buses, and trains are a few of the surfaces you may want to be careful about. One does not need to be paranoid but be aware that such surfaces could carry viruses. Wash hands often if you come in contact with such surfaces in public places.

One thing to keep in mind about using disinfectants is that you DO NOT want soap or disinfectants to go inside your body. The effect of getting disinfectants inside your body could be varied - mildly harmful as compromising your immune system to potentially serious as causing death.

Most soaps and hand sanitizers have antibacterial compounds that can kill the good bacteria in your stomach if they get inside your stomach through eating food with a sanitized hand. Good bacteria in your stomach helps overall immune health. After using soap or sanitizer, if you are going to eat with hand, make sure to wash with warm water to remove any traces of antibacterial substances on your hand.

Not touching face with unclean hands

Avoiding touching your face helps to prevent germs from getting inside your body through mouth, nose, eyes, or ears.

Social distancing and avoiding physical contacts

Social distancing, especially during times of pandemic is an important factor in getting infected as well as preventing transmission of viral and bacterial diseases. If one person is sick or suspect of being sick, not shaking hands or hugging as a way of greeting is a good practice as a precautionary. Eastern ways of greeting through bowing to each other or "namaste" greeting are something to be considered.

Wearing a mask if you need to step out you suspect you have an infection

In many Asian countries, people use masks as a practice, but this is not so in the West. Wearing masks reduces the chances of spreading any infection we may have to others. A simple way to make a DYI mask is folding a bandana or kerchief and using rubber bands on both sides and folding the ends towards the inside.

NATURAL SUBSTANCES TO BOOST IMMUNITY AND FIGHT VIRUS AND BACTERIA

GARLIC

The main active ingredient in garlic is called polysulphide allicin and is responsible primarily for its medicinal properties. This compound, allicin, formed when garlic cloves are chopped or crushed not only provides the medicinal properties but the distinct taste and smell as well.

Garlic is extremely nutritious and is a source of vitamins C and B6, along with the minerals manganese and selenium. Garlic also contains minor amounts of other minerals such as calcium, copper, potassium, phosphorous, and iron.

Allicin, the sulfur compound found in garlic has anti-microbial, anti-fungal and anti-virus capabilities. This is one of the reasons garlic was used as a remedy for plague and smallpox during medieval times. For more on garlic, please see my book titled *"Essential Spices and Herbs: Garlic"*.

GINGER

Ginger (*Zingiber officinale*) is a flowering plant whose root is widely used as a spice and traditional medicine over thousands of years in Asia. Ginger belongs to the same family as turmeric and cardamom.

Ginger is widely used in Asian cooking, especially China and India. While turmeric, which belongs to the same family as ginger is mostly used in the powder form, ginger is used as a fresh ingredient in most cooking.

Ginger has been one of the key ingredients in Asian cuisine for centuries, especially used as part of meat recipes. When dried and ground, ginger results in a white powder that is used in baking (gingerbread, cookies, crackers, cakes, etc.) and making beverages (ginger ale, ginger beer, etc.). Ginger, either powdered or fresh, can be used in teas and is an essential component of 'masala chai'.

The main bioactive active ingredient in ginger is called gingerol and it has very powerful medicinal properties. Ginger is used in several alternative/traditional medicines in the East.

While ginger has many health benefits, the one we focus on in this book is its antibacterial properties. Gingerol is considered to be effective in reducing risk infections. Some studies have shown that gingerol can inhibit the growth some of harmful bacteria. Ginger might also be effective against a virus that can cause respiratory infections called RSV virus. Studies have been conducted on the effects of gingerol against bacteria that cause gingivitis and periodontitis that have shown ginger to be effective against these. Another study has shown that fresh ginger is effective against respiratory infections. Studies have shown that ginger is also effective against fungal infections. Given these properties, consuming ginger might help improve your immunity against the potential harmful viruses and bacteria.

Beyond its antiviral and antibacterial properties, ginger helps with digestion and is a good "gut food". As I have mentioned a couple of times in this book, your gut is the seat of your body immunity and ginger can help this improve body immune system. For more on ginger, please see my book titled *"Essential Spices and Herbs: Ginger"*.

TURMERIC

Turmeric is a well-known spice in Asian cooking, especially South Asia. Turmeric comes from the root of the turmeric plant which is part of the ginger family. The turmeric root is cleaned, dried, and grinded to create the yellow turmeric powder. Turmeric is used as an herbal supplement, added to flavor food as part of curry powder or as a standalone spice, added to cosmetics, or used as a food coloring. Turmeric is also used as a skin treatment and beauty enhancer and treatment for some of the common skin infections.

Turmeric powder is bright yellow and provides a distinct yellow color to the Indian "curry powder." Turmeric has been one of the key ingredients in Asian cuisine for years.

The main active ingredient in turmeric is called curcumin, which has very powerful medicinal properties. However, there are two challenges in fully realizing the benefits of turmeric. One, the curcumin content is only about 3% of turmeric by weight. Second, curcumin is not easily absorbed by the body. Curcumin absorption can be substantially enhanced by consuming black pepper which contains piperine along with turmeric. Also, fatty foods have been proven to aid curcumin absorption as well. To consume a sufficient dosage of curcumin, a combination of curcumin/turmeric extract supplements along with a diet prepared with turmeric is recommended.

Turmeric is a rich source of many essential vitamins and minerals; it does not contain any cholesterol but is an excellent source of antioxidants and dietary fiber which helps to control bad cholesterol levels.

Turmeric's antioxidant levels are one of the highest among popular spices and herbs. For more on turmeric, please see my book titled *"Essential Spices and Herbs: Turmeric"*.

ECHINACEA

Echinacea refers to a group of flowering plans in the daisy family. Echinacea is also referred to as American coneflower. Evidence suggests many health benefits for echinacea including boosting immunity, antibiotic and antiviral properties among many others.

A number of studies have been conducted on the effectiveness of echinacea on cold-like symptoms and flu have shown that echinacea *may* prevent catching a cold and *may* also help recover quickly from flu.

Some of the echinacea varieties contain a compound known as alkalymides or alkamides which is believed to have a positive impact on the immune system. In addition to alkamides, echinacea also contains compounds such as caffeic acid, phenolic acids, rosmarinic acid, and polyacetylenes among others. All these are anti-inflammatory and antioxidant compounds that benefit human the body. Echinacea is also known to lower blood pressure and have anti-microbial properties.

As part of herbal remedies, three species of echinacea used:
- *Echinacea angustfolia*
- *Echinacea pallida*
- *Echinacea purpurea*

Echinacea roots, stems, and leaves are used for in creating teas, tinctures, extracts, and tablets. It is available to purchase over the counter or from online retailers. The typical dosage is about 1000-1500 mg per day or 7-10 mil of extract per day.

CAT'S CLAW

Cat's claw is used as a herbal supplement known for its effect on boosting the immune system. Cat's claw is a tropical vine usually found in the Amazon rainforest and south and central America. Cat's claw vine can grow up to 30 meters in height. Its bark and root have been used in South American folk medicine for centuries.

Studies have shown that consuming cat's claw over a period of several weeks has improved a person's immunity by increasing the number of white blood cells that fight infections. The anti-inflammatory properties of cat's claw can have a positive effect on improved immunity as well.

Cat's claw is mostly available in the form of tablets or extracts and the typical dosage is about 600mg-1000mg a day. Cat's claw is not recommended to be consumed if you are pregnant or breastfeeding or taken certain other medications. Please consult your doctor before taking cat's claw.

GOLDENSEAL

Goldenseal is a low, sprawling herb known under a variety of different names found mostly in the northeastern United States. Usually, a single white flower appears at the center of each set of leaves during spring. The flower develops into a red-seeded berry. Goldenseal's root has been used by the native Indian tribes for centuries as a folk medicine as an insect repellent, to heal wounds, and as a stimulant among others.

Goldenseal contains a chemical called berberine which may be attributed to its medicinal properties. Goldenseal has antifungal and antiviral properties and considered to be effective against the bacterium E.coli. Goldenseal's antibacterial properties are probably the reason native Indian's used it to treat wounds and other skin ailments.

Goldenseal may help improve digestive health which in turn can improve immunity as gastrointestinal health a key factor in the body's immune system.

Goldenseal is available in capsule form as well as cream (for topical/skin use) and tinctures (usually used for mouth ulcers). Typical dosage is 600mg-1000mg.

ALOE VERA

Aloe Vera has been used for many centuries and is considered a safe herb. Aloe Vera has antibacterial properties and considered effective against *H. Pylori* bacteria found in the digestive tract that can cause stomach ulcers.
Aloe Vera has been studied for irritable bowel syndrome (IBS) and found that it significantly improved IBS condition compared to placebo.
Aloe Vera seems to be beneficial in improving digestive health which in turn helps with improved immunity.

Aloe Vera plant may be grown in the house on your windowsill and cultivated. Typically, aloe vera is available to purchase as a gel, cream, or lotion.

EUCALYPTUS

Eucalyptus is an evergreen tree originally considered a native of Australia but currently grown all over the world.

Eucalyptus leaves contain chemical compounds (such as *eucalyptol*) that might have anti-bacterial and antifungal properties, may control blood sugar and might help pain and inflammation. In this book, we are more focused on eucalyptus anti-bacterial and anti-viral properties.

Eucalyptol (also known as *cineole*) is responsible for its effectiveness against cold and flu symptoms such as cough, nasal congestion, and headache. It may also reduce mucus build-up and help expand bronchi and bronchioles of your lungs resulting in relief for asthma.

Research studies conducted on Eucalyptol have shown both the effectiveness against cold and flu as well as asthma symptoms.

Eucalyptus is available as an essential oil, as part of cough drops, lotions, soaps, candles, chewing gum, and vapor rub. Eucalyptus is primarily used is as topical or inhalant in aromatherapy. Various different brands of eucalyptus tea are available as well.

CINNAMON

Cinnamon is also a spice used for thousands of years and is well known for its fragrance and sweetness. Used primarily in baking, cinnamon is one of the healthiest spices on earth. Cinnamon is packed with antioxidants, anti-inflammatory, anti-bacterial, and anti-fungal agents. Cinnamon is good in fighting common infections due to its anti-microbial properties. Other benefits include lower and more stabilized blood sugar levels in diabetes patients, lower cholesterol, and improved brain function. For more on cinnamon, please see my book titled *"Essential Spices and Herbs: Cinnamon"*.

ELDERBERRY

Elderberry is a flowering plant native to Europe. The berries are purple in color and tart in taste and could be poisonous if eaten raw. Elderberry is used in folk medicine for influenza, infections, and pain.

Many studies have been conducted with elderberry extracts or infusions and have shown to be effective in improving influenza, cold, fever, nasal congestion, and other flu symptoms.

Elderberry may be cooked to make jams, pies, wine, or juices. Elderberry is available commercially as gummies, teas, extracts, and lozenges.

CLOVE

Cloves are the aromatic flower buds of an evergreen tree native of South Asia. Used extensively in Indian cuisine, clove has a history of centuries of use. Clove boosts the immune system, helps with digestion and has many other benefits

LICORICE ROOT

Licorice root has been used ancient Egyptians to make medicinal concoctions as they believed that licorice could cure many diseases. In today's folk medicine, licorice root is used to treat gastrointestinal problems, improving digestion and its immune-boosting benefits. Studies have shown that licorice root extract may kill *H. Pylori* bacteria that cause stomach ulcers.

Glycyrrhizin contained in licorice root may be effective against the hepatitis C virus as found in a research study. Licorice root might also be beneficial in improving the health of the respiratory system.

HONEY

Honey is a natural sweetener, highly antioxidant, promotes sleep, soothes the throat, and heals burns and wounds. Honey combined with cinnamon is a good remedy for diabetes. Tea with honey and lemon is a remedy for cough.

APPLE CIDER VINEGAR

Apple cider vinegar has many health benefits, it promotes weight loss, lowers blood sugar and cholesterol, fights diabetes as well as cancer. Use raw unfiltered apple cider vinegar that contains "mother", strands of protein, friendly bacteria, and enzymes. Apple cider vinegar, when used in the bone broth helps to extract the nutrients contained in the bone into the broth.

Bee Pollen

Bee pollen is a mixture of flower pollen, nectar, been saliva, and wax. Bee pollen is highly nutritious and has medicinal properties. In fact, the German ministry of health recognizes bee pollen as medicine.

Bee pollen contains anti-oxidant and anti-inflammatory compounds, both of these may help in improving the body's immunity and natural healing process. Bee pollen also has antibacterial and properties and is considered effective against E.coli and salmonella. Bee pollen is available as supplements.

CBD Oils

Cannabinoids are generally immune suppressors. This means that if you are suffering from an overactive immune system, such as the case of autoimmune conditions, CBD oils may actually have benefit in chronic autoimmune diseases by reducing this intensity of such conditions and making it manageable

Curry Powder

Most of the ingredients in curry powder have anti-bacterial, antiviral, anti-fungal, and anti-microbial properties. During the middle ages, spices like turmeric, chili powder, and cinnamon were used as a food preservative due to these properties. Coriander is considered effective in treating foodborne diseases such as salmonella. All these spices have properties that make them a good choice for fighting various infections. Infections as simple as a common cold to infections such as lung and other respiratory tract infections caused by bacteria or fungi can be fought with warm curry soup.

As we have seen, ginger has antioxidant, anti-inflammatory, and anti-microbial properties, its use helps in an improved immune system. Studies have shown that ginger extract can prevent growth or even kill some of the bacteria and viruses. Studies have been conducted on the effects of gingerol against bacteria that cause gingivitis and periodontitis that have shown ginger to be effective against these. Another study has shown that fresh ginger is effective against respiratory infections. Studies have shown that ginger is also effective against fungal infections.

Curry made with curry powder, fresh ginger, garlic, and other herbs provide additional benefits in fighting bacteria and infections. Allicin, the sulfur compound found in garlic has anti-microbial, anti-fungal and anti-virus capabilities. A bowl of warm mild curry soup can be effective in 1. Preventing a cold and flu and 2. Speedy recovery in cases where the subjects of the study did catch a cold.

VITAMINS AND OTHERS

These are not necessarily natural substances as described in the previous sections. But the following are known to affect the immune system and health in a positive way

- Vitamin D. Research has shown that low Vitamin D level is linked to autoimmune diseases such as

lupus, multiple sclerosis, and rheumatoid arthritis. Vitamin D also helps reduce the risk of colds, flu, and respiratory illness
- Vitamin C. Vitamin C helps support the immune system by helping to improve overall health. Vitamin C is known to improve white blood cell levels. Vitamin C is also an antioxidant that fights free radicals.
- Vitamin B6. Vitamin B6 or Pyridoxine helps make hemoglobin, a component of the red blood cell that carries oxygen to body cells.
- Vitamin E helps fight inflections

Beyond these vitamins, sunlight (which helps with Vitamin D production), fresh air and outdoors helps boost the body's immune response and overall health.

CHAPTER 4. RECIPES FOR IMMUNE BOOSTING AND ANTIVIRAL PREPARATIONS

In olden times, the various indigenous tribes recognized the medicinal properties of herbs and spices and they used them in cooking whenever it was easier to do so. For those harder to cook or digest natural substances such as tree trunks, roots or barks different methods extracting medicinal compounds in them such as below:

- Infusions: Infusions are like tea preparations where the immune-boosting or antiviral substances are allowed to be infused in a medium (usually water). Tea preparations including some of the ones described in this book such as ginger tea can be considered as infusions. Infusions or tea preparations are usually mild in strength and a good way to stay hydrated and fasten recovery during flu and other viral infections.

- Decoctions: Decoction is a process to extract herbal or root essence by mashing the herbal root and then boiling in water to extract the herbal oils and other medicinal compounds from the herb or spice. For example, ginger root may be mashed and boiled in water to get a concentrated ginger decoction that can be taken for stomach ailments.

- Extracts: Extracts are made from the herb or root by dissolving them in water or ethanol

Today, there is no need to follow these extraction methods in your home as these herbal supplements are available in the market and in online stores in many different forms such as tablets, teas, gummies, essential oils, extracts, and tinctures.

Foods Preparations

As we have seen the easiest way to consume these healthy ingredients is to incorporate them as part of food preparations. Spices and herbs may be used as part of vegetable or meat dishes, soups, and smoothies.

IMMUNE BOOSTING RECIPES

Many of the recipes listed below contain natural ingredients that are known to have powerful antioxidant, anti-inflammatory, antibacterial and antiviral properties.

IMMUNE BOOSTING CURRY RECIPE (MEAT)

Curry powder contains many spices that are known to have benefits that help the immune system. These include chili, turmeric, coriander, cumin, cinnamon, ginger, garlic, and many others. Therefore, any curry preparation might be beneficial to your immune system. Below, two recipes are included and some tips for trying out others. If you like to get additional recipes, please see my books *"Introduction to CURRY"* and *"A Beginner's Guide to Cooking with Spices"*.

The recipe below for chicken curry is a sample recipe that can be adapted to make several different versions including a non-meat version as explained in the recipe notes below.

Ingredients

- 2 lbs. chicken thighs and legs bone-in
- 1-2 tsp of mild curry powder, depending on your tolerance on spice
- 2 tbsp coriander powder
- ½ tsp turmeric powder
- 2 medium onion chopped
- 2-3 tsp coconut oil
- ½ tsp garam masala (optional)
- 1-2 jalapenos slit (optional)
- ½ tsp cumin powder

- 1 inch fresh ginger grated
- 6-10 cloves of garlic chopped
- 2 medium potatoes peeled and cut
- 2-3 medium tomatoes sliced
- Salt to taste
- ½ -1 can of chicken broth/bone broth (depending on the amount gravy desired)
- ½ cup cilantro chopped

Method

1. Sprinkle ½ tsp curry powder, turmeric, and ¼ tsp salt on cut chicken. Mix well and keep it aside for 30 minutes.
2. In a separate pan, heat oil, sauté onions, garlic, ginger, and optional jalapenos until onions become translucent.
3. Add remaining curry powder, and also the other spices and mix for 1-2 minutes so the spices are cooked. Make sure not to burn spices.
4. Add potatoes, mix well and cook covered for 5 minutes or until potatoes are tender. Now add chicken and mix it on high heat for one minute so that any raw spices sticking to the chicken as marinade gets fried in oil and also the chicken pieces are well coated with spices and herbs. Add tomato, cover, and cook for 15-20 minutes on low flame. Add enough chicken broth for the desired thickness. Stir occasionally.
5. Once the chicken and potatoes are cooked, add cilantro and stir. Add salt to taste. Switch off the heat and keep it covered for 1-2 minutes before serving.

Serve with rice or bread.

Recipe Notes:

1. This same recipe could be made in ½ the time by using an instant pot or electric pressure cooker to cook potatoes and chicken. If you are using an instant pot, first saute in the pot and then close the lid and cook for 10 minutes or poultry setting.
2. You could make the recipe without potatoes and only chicken. The same steps would work
3. Instead of potato or in addition to potato you may use one or more of the following vegetables:
    a. Carrots
    b. Italian squash
    c. Bell pepper – green, red or yellow
    d. Green plantain

    Different combination of these vegetables will get you slightly different chicken curry each time

4. Depending on your spice tolerance level, you can increase or decrease the amount of spices used.
5. The amount of chicken broth added will determine how thick the curry soup will come out.
6. You can make the same curry without chicken to prepare a non-meat recipe.

IMMUNE BOOSTING CURRY RECIPE (VEGAN)

Basic Ingredients

- 2 medium potatoes peeled and cut into 1-inch cubes
- ½ head of cauliflower washed and cut into small pieces (same size as the potatoes)
- 2 teaspoon oil
- 1 medium onion sliced
- 1 teaspoon curry powder
- 1-2 medium tomatoes chopped
- ½ teaspoon salt (or to taste)
- ¼ cup fresh cilantro chopped
- ½ cup vegetable broth

Optional Ingredients
- 1-2 jalapenos sliced (seeds out/in)
- 2-3 cloves of garlic crushed
- ½ inch ginger root chopped into fine pieces

Method

1. Heat oil in a medium non-stick pan and crackle optional cumin seeds.
2. Add onions, and optional garlic, ginger, and jalapenos. Stir until onion becomes translucent.
3. Add turmeric, black pepper, and optional curry powder, stir for 1-2 minutes.
4. Add chopped tomatoes, potatoes, and cauliflower, mix well and then add vegetable broth and mix
5. Bring to a boil
6. Cover and simmer for 10-15 minutes, or until the potatoes and cauliflower are cooked.

7. Switch off the heat and add the cilantro and salt.

Mix well and serve hot as a side dish with rice or bread.

Recipe Notes:

1. There are many optional ingredients listed, one could use all of them or pick and choose based on your taste.
2. The jalapenos vary in their heat level. If you choose to use them, you can take the seeds out to reduce the heat.

SPICY BONE BROTH (CHICKEN)

This is a spicy version of the previous chicken bone broth. This spicy broth immediately helps with congestion, cold, flu, sore throat, and other ailments due to infections. This broth also is healing and easy for your gut besides all the long-term health benefits that come with regular consumption of these bone broth and healing spices.

Basic Ingredients:

- 4 lb. chicken bones – any combination of wings, necks, and feet.
- 4 celery sticks cut into 1 inch pieces
- 3 medium tomatoes chopped
- 1 bell pepper cut into pieces (any color)
- 1 large onion peeled and quartered

- 1 pound (2-3 medium) carrots washed cut into pieces
- 1 gallon water
- 2 tablespoon raw unfiltered apple cider vinegar
- Salt to taste (if you must or avoid salt)

Spices & Herbs

- 2 tsp turmeric powder
- 1 tsp cumin powder or 1tsp cumin seeds
- 1 tsp coriander powder
- 1 tsp cayenne powder
- 2 tsp fenugreek seeds
- ½ cup parsley chopped
- ½ cup cilantro chopped
- ½ cup rosemary
- 3-4 garlic cloves crushed
- 3-4 whole cloves
- 2 inch ginger peeled and grated
- 5-6 black peppercorns or ½ tsp pepper powder
- 1-2 bay leaves
- 1-2 Jalapeño pepper slit (optional)

Method

1. In a medium a pan, heat oil, crackle cumin seeds, and fenugreek seeds. Add onions, crushed garlic, ginger, jalapeño peppers

2. Sauté for 2-3 minutes or until onions become translucent. Add all the spices (cayenne, cumin, turmeric, coriander, cloves, bay leaves, and pepper powder) and sauté for another 2-3 minutes so the

spices are blended well and sufficiently roasted (make sure not to burn the spices).

3. Transfer the spice mix into a large pot (add some water to wash out any remaining spice mix from the pan and pour it into the large pot)

4. Add all chicken bones and vegetables into a large crock-pot and add water, apple cider vinegar and bring to a boil.

5. Lower the heat, simmer covered for 24-48 hours.

6. Once the bones and vegetables are cooked, strain the broth into a large bowl

7. Add salt to taste, add some chopped fresh herbs of your choice, and serve warm.

8. Refrigerate any remaining broth

ANTIVIRAL AND ANTIBACTERIAL RECIPES

These recipes are good to boost immunity as well as fight cold or flu symptoms.

These drinks keep you hydrated as well as boost your body's firepower against viral, fungal, or bacterial infections.

TURMERIC TEA WITH GINGER

This is a simple tea (does not use any regular tea bag/leaves) that contain just the wonder spices turmeric, ginger, and black pepper. This is an anti-inflammatory drink that can also provide immediate relief from cold, flu, upset stomach, or nausea.

Ingredients

- ½ - 2 teaspoon turmeric powder or ½ inch – 2 inch long fresh turmeric root, grated
- ½ inch – 1 inch fresh ginger, grated/ sliced
- 1 teaspoon honey (or as much to sweeten the tea to your taste)
- Pinch of freshly ground black pepper or pepper powder
- 1-2 cups of water

Method

1. Put the turmeric, ground pepper and ginger in a cup or pot and add one spoon of water, mix and make it a paste.
2. Boil 1-2 cups of water and add to the turmeric & ginger paste. Mix it well.
3. Strain out the ginger/turmeric pieces. Let it cool for a couple of minutes and add honey and enjoy warm.

HOT TURMERIC MILK

This is an alternative version of turmeric and ginger tea with additional spices and milk. This has all the benefits of ginger turmeric tea and more and is a common drink grandmothers and mothers make in India as a remedy for flu and cold symptoms.

Ingredients

- ½ - 2 teaspoon turmeric powder or ½ inch – 2-inch-long fresh turmeric root, sliced
- ½-1inch fresh ginger, grated or thinly sliced
- ¼ teaspoon ground cardamom (or 2-3 cardamom pods crushed)
- 1 brown sugar (or as much to sweeten to your taste)
- 1 pinch of freshly ground black pepper or pepper powder
- 1 pinch of ground cloves (or 2-3 crushed cloves - optional)
- 1-2 cups of milk of your choice (regular, coconut or almond)

Method

1. Mix turmeric, cardamom, black pepper, and cloves in a bowl.
2. Boil 1-2 cups of milk and add the turmeric mixture and mix well. Careful not to boil over.
3. Strain out any lumps if need be. Let it cool for a couple of minutes enjoy as is or add sugar and enjoy warm.

GREEN TEA WITH TURMERIC & GINGER

This is another remedy for cold and flu symptoms. Green tea has more antioxidants than regular black tea. Green tea combined with turmeric and ginger is a great combination.

Ingredients

- ½ - 2 teaspoon turmeric powder or ½ inch – 2 inch long fresh turmeric
- ½ inch – 1 inch fresh ginger grated/sliced
- 1 teaspoon honey (or as much to sweeten the tea to your taste)
- 1 pinch of freshly ground black pepper or pepper powder
- 1-2 cups of green tea.

Method

1. Process all the ingredients in a blender until smooth.
2. Add the hot green tea, mix well.
3. Filter if needed. Add honey and enjoy.

Recipe note:

If using fresh turmeric root, either grind it as part of the rest of the ingredients or boil the root in 1-2 cups of water and green tea for 5 minutes on low heat. Then add pepper and honey once it cools down.

GINGER AND LEMON TEA

Ingredients

- ½ inch – 1 inch fresh ginger grated or crushed
- ½ tsp lemon juice
- 1 tsp honey

Method

1. Boil 2 cups of water in a saucepan.
2. Add ginger and let it boil for 2-3 minutes.
3. Remove from heat and add lemon. Add honey once it is sufficiently cooled down. Enjoy warm.

This drink is good for nausea. Drink as often as needed.

GARLIC TEA WITH GINGER AND LEMON

In this tea, we introduce garlic which is a very healthy spice (or vegetable-based on how you look at it) into the mix.

Ingredients

- 1-2 cloves of garlic crushed
- ½ inch fresh ginger grated or thinly sliced
- 1 tsp honey (or as much to sweeten the tea to your taste)
- 1 tsp lemon juice
- 2 cups of water
- pinch of black pepper powder (optional)

Method

1. Boil 2 cups of water and add crushed garlic and ginger and let it boil for 1 minute.
2. Add optional pepper.
3. Switch off the heat and let it sit for 20 minutes.
4. Strain out the ginger/garlic pieces. Let it cool for a couple of minutes
5. Add honey and lemon juice and enjoy warm.

This drink is good for digestion, fighting cold/flu, clearing nasal congestion and sore throat, etc.

Recipe note: Optionally 2 tsp apple cider vinegar also may be added to the boiled water along with the rest of the ingredients.

GINGER *RASAM*

Rasam is a light, thin soup preparation in south India, Sri Lanka, and other southeast Asian countries. *Rasam* is usually served with rice or can be taken as is especially if you are under fighting cold, nasal congestion, and other flu symptoms. There are many variations of *rasam*. The one given below is simple and especially effective to relieve flu symptoms.

Ingredients

- 1-2 tsp rasam powder
- 1 inch fresh ginger grated or thinly sliced
- 6 cloves garlic
- 5 cups of water
- ½ tsp black pepper powder
- 2 tomatoes chopped
- 1 tsp mustard seeds
- ¼ tsp asafoetida
- 2 tbsp tamarind pulp
- 1 spring curry leaves
- ¼ cup cilantro
- 2 tbsp coconut oil/vegetable oil
- Salt to taste
- ½ tsp sugar (optional)

Method

1. Heat oil in a deep pan, crackle mustard seeds, add curry leaves and asafetida. Saute for 30 seconds.
2. Add rasam powder and saute for 1 minute

3. Add chopped up tomatoes and mix well. Saute for another minute or until tomatoes soften.
4. Add tamarind pulp, salt, and optional sugar. Bring it to a boil.
5. Allow it to simmer for 5 minutes or until tomatoes are cooked.
6. Add chopped up cilantro. Switch off the heat and serve warm.

Recipe Notes:

1. Various different brands of rasam powder is available to buy in many south Asian stores. If you can't find rasam powder, follow the simple recipe below:
    a. Roast 1 tsp whole black pepper, 2-3 red chilies, 1 tsp cumin, 6 cloves, ½ coriander seeds
    b. Grind them in a food processor.
    c. Increase the proportion if you want to make additional batches
2. Some rasam powder may include roasted split lentils. You can add a couple of tablespoons of split lentils to the above recipe to make rasam powder
3. In some rasam preparations, ½ cup of cooked split lentil is added. But it is not needed if you are preparing it as a cold remedy.

HYDRATING DRINK RECIPES

SIMPLE LEMON WATER

There are several ways of making lemon water. How much lemon juice one uses is a personal preference. Lime juice may be used instead of lemon juice. In some cases, salt or sugar is added to the lemon drink to enhance the taste.

Irrespective of how it is made (the amount of juice, lime or lemon or salt or sugar is added), lemon water is a great way to hydrate your body. Lemon water has vitamin-C and antioxidants. A glass of warm (or room temperature) lemon water helps in digestion and detoxification. Lemon water is also considered to be good for skin as the antioxidants, especially in lemon, helps in rejuvenating the skin. When you have flu or other virus infections, lemon water is a good choice to keep you hydrated.

Several ways to make

1. Juice (or squeeze) ½ lemon and add the juice to about 8 once (a tall cup) or water (cold or room temperature depending on preference). Mix well. This is the simplest one

2. Like in step 1 make the lemon/lime water. Add ½ teaspoon Himalayan salt (or sea salt) and mix well. This is a very refreshing drink after exercise or on a hot day.

3. As in step 1 make the lemon/lime water. Add 1-2 teaspoon brown sugar. Mix well until the sugar dissolves completely. Some people prefer sweet lemon drink.

LEMON WATER WITH GINGER AND MINT

As in the previous recipe, make about 2 tall glasses of lemon/lime water. Crush 1 teaspoon ginger and 1 teaspoon mint leaves in a mortar. Add to the lemon water, add 1-2 teaspoon brown sugar (optional) and mix well. Strain the contents into a jug. Refrigerate until ready to serve.

LEMON WATER WITH CUCUMBER AND MINT LEAVES

Add 1 washed and sliced cucumber, ¼ cup mint leaves, one lemon washed and sliced, one teaspoon grated ginger to 2 liters of water. Mix well and refrigerate overnight. Drink 1 cup first thing in the morning. This drink helps digestion, increased metabolism, helps rejuvenate the body (including skin) and nourishes and hydrates the body besides boosting immunity. Good source of vitamins A, B, and C. Due to improved metabolism, some consumers of this drink have reported weight loss after consuming this link regularly before breakfast.

FRUIT-INFUSED WATER

1. Slice a couple of strawberries and add them into a pitcher of water. Add a few mint leaves. Mix well and let it sit for 4-6 hours.

2. Wash and slice a medium orange and add it into a pitcher of water. Mix well and set aside for at least 4 hours before using.

3. Watermelon and herbs. Cut a cup of watermelon pieces in a pitcher of water add some herbs of your choice (mint, basil, rosemary). Set it aside for about 2-3 hours before using it.

GINGER ALE

Ingredients

- 1 cup ginger, peeled and sliced

- 2-3 cups of water
- ½ -1 cup brown sugar
- 1 teaspoon freshly squeezed lemon juice

Method

1. Add ginger to boiling water and simmer it for 10-15 minutes. Stir well.
2. Add sugar and let it fully dissolve.
3. Put off the heat and let it sit until warm.
4. Strain the ginger pieces. Add lemon juice and stir. Pour the contents into a glass jar and refrigerate it.

The mixture may be used as-is (one spoon at a time) for nausea and indigestion or heartburn. You can also add 4-5 teaspoons of this mixture into a glass of club soda and drink.

BUTTERMILK DRINK

This is a well-known drink in South India, especially during summertime. In its simplest form, 1 cup buttermilk and 1 cup water are combined with one tbsp grated ginger and finely chopped jalapeño peppers (with or without seeds depending on your heat level) pulse it in a blender and add some cilantro or curry leaves and salt to taste.

Below is a bit more elaborate way to make buttermilk drink

Ingredients

- 2 cups of buttermilk
- 2 cups of filtered water

- 1 teaspoon minced ginger
- ½ -1 jalapeño seeds removed and minced
- ¼ cup cilantro leaves finely chopped
- 1 teaspoon coconut (or vegetable) oil
- ½ teaspoon mustard seeds
- 1 spring curry leaves
- ½ teaspoon turmeric powder (optional)
- 1 teaspoon lemon juice (optional)
- salt to taste

Method

1. Combine buttermilk, water, lemon juice, ginger, jalapeño, and cilantro in a blender and blend for about 15 seconds.
2. Heat oil in a pan and crackle mustard seeds and add curry leaves. Add optional turmeric powder. Mix for about 30 seconds. Add it to the blended buttermilk mixture. Mix and serve.

Buttermilk drinks are common on a hot day in South India. This drink (with turmeric option) is a good remedy for cold/flu and also for hydrating during nausea or diarrhea.

APPLE CIDER VINEGAR DRINK

Ingredients:

- 1 tablespoon apple cider vinegar (raw unfiltered)
- 2 cups of water
- ½ tbsp lime juice
- dash of cinnamon powder

Method

Mix together drink on an empty stomach daily. This drink helps promote weight loss, reduce cholesterol, fight diabetes, and promote overall wellness.

ANTI-INFLAMMATORY RECIPES

Inflammation plays an important role in the natural healing process in the human body. It helps to defend harmful invaders in our body such as bacteria that cause infection. Inflammation also helps the body carry out wound repair. Without inflammation, these foreign invaders could cause damage to our bodies and ultimately kill us.

While short term, controlled inflammation is beneficial, it can become a major problem when it becomes chronic, such as arthritis. Chronic inflammation plays a major role in many serious health conditions such as heart disease, cancer, Alzheimer's, and other various degenerative conditions.

Therefore, it is very important that inflammation is contained, and chronic inflammation condition is fought with either medicine, supplements, or through foods or a combination of both in order to reduce or prevent it from happening. Anti-inflammatory foods help the body to prevent chronic inflammation help boost its natural inflammation process that helps defend infections and prevent autoimmune conditions.

The recipes below use natural herbs and spices such as turmeric, ginger, cinnamon, and other anti-inflammatory ingredients.

GREEN SMOOTHIE WITH GARLIC, GINGER, AND TURMERIC

A power-packed, extremely healthy smoothie that combines the goodness of greens with medicinal spices.

Ingredients

- ½ inch – 2 inches long fresh cleaned and sliced turmeric root
- ½ inch – 1 inch fresh ginger peeled
- 1 clove garlic
- 1 tsp honey (optional to taste)
- 1 pinch of freshly ground black pepper or pepper powder
- 1 cup of kale
- 1 cup spinach
- 1-2 kiwi peeled
- ½ cup blueberries
- ½ cup sliced cucumber (optional)
- ¼ avocado (optional)
- 3-4 mint leaves
- 1-2 cup filtered water (coconut water may be used as well)
- ½ cup ice

Method

Process all the ingredients in a blender until smooth. Blueberries may be substituted by blackberries depending on your liking. Serves 3-4.

By mixing and matching the "green" ingredients, you may try a couple of different green smoothies. You can substitute cucumber with broccoli.

GOLDEN YELLOW SMOOTHIE

Coconut oil is known to have many benefits and it also helps the absorption of curcumin from turmeric.

Ingredients

- ½ - 2 spoon turmeric powder or ½ inch – 2 inches long fresh cleaned and sliced turmeric root
- ½ inch – 1 inch fresh ginger grated or thinly sliced
- 1 tsp honey (optional to taste)
- 1 tsp coconut oil
- 1 carrot washed and cut into pieces
- 1 mango peeled and sliced
- 1 cup Orange or Mango Juice
- ½ cup ice

Method

Process all the ingredients in a blender until smooth.

VERY BERRY SMOOTHIE

Berries are superfoods with many benefits including fighting cancer, anti-aging by keeping your brain young. Fights Alzheimer's and Parkinson's.

Ingredients

- ½ inch – 1 inch fresh ginger grated or thinly sliced
- 1 tsp honey (optional to taste)
- ½ cup blueberries
- ½ cup blackberries
- ½ cup raspberries
- ½ cup strawberries
- 1 cup 2% milk or low-fat yogurt
- ½ cup ice

Method

Process all the ingredients in a blender until smooth.

VEGAN BROTH

This is a simple broth that provides healing and helps with minor ailments such as cold and flu. This is fully vegan and contains nutrients from a number of vegetables and herbs.

Ingredients

- 2-3 celery sticks cut into inch pieces
- 3 medium tomatoes chopped
- 1 bell pepper cut into pieces
- 1 large onion peeled and cut into pieces
- 1 pound (2-3 medium) carrots washed cut into pieces
- 1 cup kale
- 1 medium beetroot washed and cut into pieces
- ½ cup parsley chopped
- ½ cup cilantro chopped
- 3-4 garlic cloves crushed

- 3-4 whole cloves
- 5-6 black peppercorns or ½ tsp pepper powder
- 1-2 bay leaves
- 1 gallon water
- Salt to taste (if you must or avoid salt)

Method

1. Add everything to a large pot. Bring to a boil

2. Lower the heat, simmer covered for about 1 hr. Stir occasionally

3. Once the vegetables are cooked, strain the broth into a large bowl

4. Add salt to taste, add some chopped fresh herbs of your choice and serve warm.

5. Refrigerate any remaining broth

6. The strained vegetables are pretty good and can be eaten separately or pureed in a blender used.

SPICY VEGAN BROTH

This is a spicy version of the vegan broth that immediately helps with congestion, cold, flu, sore throat, and other ailments due to infections. Like the non-spicy version, this broth also is healing and easy for your gut. The antioxidants and anti-inflammatory compounds in turmeric and ginger make this broth even healthier.

Ingredients: Veggies

- 2-3 celery sticks cut into inch pieces
- 3 medium tomatoes chopped
- 1 bell green pepper cut into pieces
- 1 red bell pepper cut into pieces
- ¼ of a medium red cabbage chopped
- 1 large onion peeled and cut into 1-inch cubes
- ½ cup chopped onion (for sautéing)
- 1 pound (2-3 medium) carrots washed cut into pieces
- 1 cup kale
- 1 medium beetroot washed and cut into pieces

Ingredients – spices and herbs
- ½ cup parsley chopped
- ½ cup cilantro chopped
- 3-4 garlic cloves crushed
- 3-4 whole cloves
- 5-6 black peppercorns or ½ tsp pepper powder
- 1-2 bay leaves
- 1 inch ginger finely chopped
- 2 tsp turmeric powder or 2 inch fresh root
- 2 jalapeño pepper sliced lengthwise (seed in or out depending on your heat tolerance)

- ½ tsp cayenne powder
- ½ tsp cumin powder
- 1 gallon water
- salt to taste (if you must or avoid salt)
- 1 tsp coconut or vegetable oil

Method

1. In a medium pan, heat oil and add onions, crushed garlic, ginger, jalapeño peppers.

2. Sauté for 2-3 minutes or until onions become translucent. Add all the spices (cayenne, cumin, turmeric, cloves, bay leaves pepper powder) and sauté for another 2-3 minutes so the spices are blended well (make sure not to burn the spices).

3. Transfer the spice mix into a large pot (add some water to wash out any remaining spice mix from the pan and pour it into the large pot)

4. Add all the vegetables into the pot and add water, bring to a boil.

5. Lower the heat, simmer covered for about 1 hr. Stir occasionally

6. Once the vegetables are cooked, strain the broth into a large bowl

7. Add salt to taste, add some chopped fresh herbs of your choice, and serve warm.

8. Refrigerate any remaining broth

The strained-out vegetables are also nutritious and may be consumed separately.

EASY BONE BROTH (CHICKEN)

This is one of the easiest ways to make bone broth. I make it out of the carcass from the rotisserie chicken bought from the departmental store. I remove all the meat and use it as a regular meal for the family and use the entire carcass (without the skins – but skins may be used as well if you prefer) for the bone broth

Ingredients

- Chicken carcass from a full rotisserie chicken – skin and fat optional
- 4 celery sticks cut into 1-inch pieces
- 3 medium tomatoes chopped
- 1 bell pepper cut into pieces (any color)
- 1 large onion peeled and quartered
- 1 pound (2-3 medium) carrots washed cut into pieces
- ½ cup parsley chopped
- ½ cup cilantro chopped
- 3-4 garlic cloves crushed
- 3-4 whole cloves
- 2 inch ginger peeled and grated
- 5-6 black peppercorns or ½ tsp pepper powder
- 1-2 bay leaves
- 1 Jalapeño pepper slit (optional)
- 1 gallon water
- Salt to taste (if you must or avoid salt)

Method

1. Add everything to a large pot. Bring to a boil

2. Lower the heat, simmer covered for about 2-3 hrs.

3. Once the vegetables are fully cooked, strain the broth into a large bowl using a mesh strainer.

4. Add salt to taste, add some chopped fresh herbs of your choice, and serve warm.

5. Refrigerate any remaining broth

Recipe Notes:

1. The strained vegetables are pretty good and can be eaten after removing all the bone pieces.

2. A slow cooker or pressure cooker may be used for cooking. A pressure cooker will reduce the cooking time if you are in a hurry.

3. You can make this broth a meal by making it a soup. For making it a soup – add ½ cup split lentils, ½ cup brown or white rice to the pot. Use a mesh strainer to strain so the cooked rice and lentils pass through. Add some of the vegetables back and enjoy it especially when you are recovering from illness or when you don't feel like having a full meal but something filling and nutritious.

BEEF BONE BROTH

Ingredients:

- 4 lb. beef bones – a mix of marrow bones, knuckle bones, short ribs
- 4 celery sticks cut into 1 inch pieces
- 3 medium tomatoes chopped
- 1 large onion peeled and quartered
- 1 pound (2-3 medium) carrots washed cut into pieces
- 3-4 beets with leaves. Leaves chopped. Beets peeled and cut into pieces
- 2 inch ginger piece peeled and grated
- 3-4 cloves of garlic
- 1 gallon water
- Salt to taste
- Pepper to taste
- ½ cup cilantro
- ½ cup parsley
- 2 tablespoon apple cider vinegar

Method

1. Add everything to a large pot. Bring to a boil

2. Using a slotted spoon, remove any foam or scum that rises to the top and continue to skim the top until the broth is clear.

3. Reduce the heat and let it simmer for one hour. Remove any remaining fat or foam rising to the top

4. Cover and simmer the broth for 18-24 hrs.

5. Switch off the heat. Strain the broth into a large bowl using a mesh strainer.

6. Add salt to taste, add some chopped fresh herbs of your choice, and serve warm.

SPICY BEEF BONE BROTH

This is a spicy version of the previous beef bone broth.

Basic Ingredients:

- 4 lb. beef bones – a mix of marrow bones, knuckle bones, short ribs
- 4 celery stalks cut into 1 inch pieces
- 3 medium tomatoes chopped
- 1 bell pepper cut into pieces (any color)
- 1 large onion peeled and quartered
- 1 pound (2-3 medium) carrots washed cut into pieces
- 1 gallon water
- 3 tablespoon raw unfiltered apple cider vinegar
- Salt to taste (if you must or avoid salt)
- 2 tsp coconut oil

Spices & Herbs

- 2 tsp turmeric powder
- 1 tsp cumin powder or 1tsp cumin seeds
- 1 tsp coriander powder
- 1 tsp cayenne powder
- 2 tsp fenugreek seeds

- ½ cup parsley chopped
- ½ cup cilantro chopped
- ½ cup rosemary
- 3-4 garlic cloves crushed
- 3-4 whole cloves
- 2 inch ginger peeled and grated
- 5-6 black peppercorns or ½ tsp pepper powder
- 1-2 bay leaves
- 1-2 Jalapeño pepper slit (optional)

Method

1. In a medium pan, heat oil, crackle cumin seeds, and fenugreek seeds. Add onions, crushed garlic, ginger, and jalapeño peppers

2. Sauté for 2-3 minutes or until onions become translucent. Add all the spices (cayenne, cumin, turmeric, coriander, cloves, bay leaves, and pepper powder) and sauté for another 2-3 minutes so the spices are blended well and sufficiently roasted (make sure not to burn the spices).

3. Transfer the spice mix into a large pot (add some water to wash out any remaining spice mix from the pan and pour it into the large pot)

4. Add all chicken bones and vegetables into a large crock-pot and add water, bring to a boil.

5. Add vinegar. Lower the heat, simmer covered for 24-48 hours.

6. Once the bones and vegetables are cooked, strain the broth into a large bowl

7. Add salt to taste, add some chopped fresh herbs of your choice, and serve warm.

8. Refrigerate any remaining broth

FINAL NOTES ON RECIPES

While there are many other anti-inflammatory and immune-boosting recipes available, I have chosen these recipes carefully based on the following:

- They include one or more immune-boosting, anti-inflammatory, and anti-viral ingredients
- They are based on fresh ingredients, no processed, canned or preserved ingredients are used
- They use medicinal spices and herbs
- A number of these recipes are drinks and others are sauce based. The reason is that during the flu, in addition to the anti-viral components, it is also important to keep the body hydrated and drink a lot of fluids. These recipes deliver much-needed fluids to the body and help prevent or fight the virus and recover from the illness quickly.
- These recipes may be adapted to your taste, availability of ingredients, and how much time you want to spend on preparing them.
- If you are new to spices and herbs, make sure to check you can tolerate them before starting to use them. If you are allergic to or sensitive to some of the spices, you may skip them in the preparation.

- Most of these recipes should be easy on the tummy and boost the digestive system, which is key to immune response. However, if any particular ingredient does not sit with your tummy, avoid it.

IMMUNE BOOSTING SUPPLEMENTS

While most foods described in this book may be used in cooking, some of the brain healthy foods are best taken as supplements. Supplements are available to buy in many online stores such as Amazon and other specialty and nutritional stores. Below are some of the brain-boosting supplements, their typical dosage and popular brands (as per this author):

Turmeric: Turmeric supplements are one of the most popular natural supplements and are usually labeled as "turmeric curcumin" and often includes other ingredients such as black pepper to help absorption and bioavailability. The typical dosage is 1000mg to 1500mg per day. Some turmeric supplements include ginger. Some of the popular brands are Nature Made, Vimerson Health, Bio Shawartz, Physician's CHOICE, NatureWise, and many others.

Garlic: Garlic supplements are widely available and many claim odor control where garlic odor is suppressed. The typical dosage is 1000mg to 2000mg per day. Some of the popular brands are BRI Nutrition, Puritan's Pride, Kyolic, Nature's Bounty, and Sundown. Garlic supplement is also available as garlic oil soft gels.

Ginger: Ginger supplements are available as standalone or combined with turmeric. The typical dosage is 1000mg per day. Popular brands are Vimerson Health, Puritan's pride and Nature's way.

Echinacea: Echinacea supplements available as standalone with goldenseal or with elderberry. The typical dosage is 1000-1500 mg per day. Popular brands include Nature's way, Nature's bounty, Herbal Secrets, and NOW

Goldenseal: Goldenseal is available in tablet form. The typical dosage is 600-1000mg. Popular brands include Nature's way, Herbal Secrets, NOW, and Nutricost

Aloe Vera: Aloe Vera is mainly available as gel, lotion or juice. Gel and lotion are for skin and hair while juice may be consumed orally. There are a number of different brands available on Amazon.com. Please read the label before using it.

Cinnamon: Cinnamon supplements are available as capsules. The typical dosage is 1200mg-1500mg. Popular brands include NutriFlair, Pure Natural, Nature's Bounty, Nature's Nutrition among others.

Cat's Claw: Cat's claw is available as capsules and extracts in the supplement market. The typical dosage is 500mg – 1500mg. Popular brands include NOW, Swanson, and Nature's Way among others.

Licorice: Licorice root supplements are available as tablets, tea, and liquid extract. The recommended dosage is 600mg-900mg. The popular brands include Himalaya organic, NOW, Yogi, and DGL.

Eucalyptus: Eucalyptus is available in the supplement market primarily as an essential oil to be used in diffusers and aromatherapy. Some of the popular brands include Handcraft Blend, Ola Prima, and Cliganic.

Elderberry: Elderberry is available as gummies, capsules and extract. The typical dosage is 600mg- 2000mg. Popular brands include Nature's Way, Havasu Nutrition, Bio Schwartz and others.

While many of the above supplements are available as capsules, some are available in teabag form or in powder form. You can make tea by steeping these tea bags in hot/boiling water for about 3-6 minutes. If you are getting powder, these powders may be added to smoothies to convert an ordinary smoothie to an immune-boosting one.

Note About Dietary Supplement Market:

The dietary supplement market is not as regulated as the regular drug market. There are also numerous companies offering different supplements with wide-ranging and often wild claims. It is important to stick with trusted brands if you choose to go for supplements. If you are purchasing online, make sure that it is from a trusted brand. My recommendation is to start shopping supplements by going to one of the larger/reputed general nutritional stores first before starting to shop online. If a reputed store is willing to bet their reputation on the supplement, that provides one proof point. Also, you get to talk to someone at the store.

Always, consult a physician if you plan to take supplements long term or you are pregnant or breast-feeding.

Also, note that the brands listed for supplements are some of the known or popular brands at the time writing this book. This may change in the future and the author is no way endorsing any of the brands. Please also note that some supplement or a combination of supplement works better for you while others not. Please do your research before buying any dietary supplements.

DISCLAIMER

This book details the author's personal experiences in using Indian spices, the information contained in the public domain as well as the author's opinion. The author is not licensed as a doctor, nutritionist, or chef. The author is providing this book and its contents on an "as is" basis and makes no representations or warranties of any kind with respect to this book or its contents. The author disclaims all such representations and warranties, including for example warranties of merchantability and educational or medical advice for a particular purpose. In addition, the author does not represent or warrant that the information accessible via this book is accurate, complete, or current. The statements made about products and services have not been evaluated by the US FDA or any equivalent organization in other countries.

The author will not be liable for damages arising out of or in connection with the use of this book or the information contained within. This is a comprehensive limitation of liability that applies to all damages of any kind, including (without limitation) compensatory; direct, indirect or consequential damages; loss of data, income or profit; loss of or damage to property and claims of third parties. It is understood that this book is not intended as a substitute for consultation with a licensed medical or a culinary professional. Before starting any lifestyle changes, it is recommended that you consult a licensed professional to ensure that you are doing what's best for your situation. The use of this book implies your acceptance of this disclaimer.

Thank You

Thank you for purchasing this book. If you enjoyed this book or found it useful, I would greatly appreciate it if you could post a short review on Amazon. I read all the reviews and your feedback will help me to make this book even better.

APPENDIX I. SOURCES AND REFERENCES

This book was written based on the author's personal experience with superfoods and spices as well as information from a wide range of sources. Some of the key sources are outlined below, in case the reader would like to read more details about natural antivirals and antibiotics.

Garlic

Preventing the common cold with a garlic supplement: a double-blind, placebo-controlled survey.

https://www.ncbi.nlm.nih.gov/pubmed/11697022

Supplementation with aged garlic extract improves both NK and γδ-T cell function and reduces the severity of cold and flu symptoms: a randomized, double-blind, placebo-controlled nutrition intervention.

https://www.ncbi.nlm.nih.gov/pubmed/22280901

Cat's claw

Persistent response to pneumococcal vaccine in individuals supplemented with a novel water soluble extract of Uncaria tomentosa, C-Med-100.

https://www.ncbi.nlm.nih.gov/pubmed/11515716

Enhanced DNA repair, immune function and reduced toxicity of C-MED-100, a novel aqueous extract from Uncaria tomentosa.

https://www.ncbi.nlm.nih.gov/pubmed/10687868

Anti-inflammatory activity of two different extracts of Uncaria tomentosa (Rubiaceae).

https://www.ncbi.nlm.nih.gov/pubmed/12065162

Echinacea

Immunomodulation with echinacea - a systematic review of controlled clinical trials.

https://www.ncbi.nlm.nih.gov/pubmed/23195946

Evaluation of echinacea for the prevention and treatment of the common cold: a meta-analysis.

https://www.ncbi.nlm.nih.gov/pubmed/17597571

Immune enhancing effects of Echinacea purpurea root extract by reducing regulatory T cell number and function.

https://www.ncbi.nlm.nih.gov/pubmed/24868871

Enhancement of innate and adaptive immune functions by multiple Echinacea species.

https://www.ncbi.nlm.nih.gov/pubmed/17887935

Eucalyptus

Efficacy of cineole in patients suffering from acute bronchitis: a placebo-controlled double-blind trial.

https://www.ncbi.nlm.nih.gov/pubmed/24261680

Therapy for acute nonpurulent rhinosinusitis with cineole: results of a double-blind, randomized, placebo-controlled trial.

https://www.ncbi.nlm.nih.gov/pubmed/15064633

Anti-inflammatory activity of 1.8-cineol (eucalyptol) in bronchial asthma: a double-blind placebo-controlled trial.

https://www.ncbi.nlm.nih.gov/pubmed/12645832

Immune-modifying and antimicrobial effects of Eucalyptus oil and simple inhalation devices.

https://www.ncbi.nlm.nih.gov/pubmed/20359267

Ginger

Antibacterial effect of *Allium sativum* cloves and *Zingiber officinale* rhizomes against multiple-drug resistant clinical pathogens

https://www.ncbi.nlm.nih.gov/pmc/articles/PMC3609356/

Inhibitory effect of Allium sativum and Zingiber officinale extracts on clinically important drug resistant pathogenic bacteria https://www.ncbi.nlm.nih.gov/pmc/articles/PMC3418209/

Fresh ginger (Zingiber officinale) has anti-viral activity against human respiratory syncytial virus in human respiratory tract cell lines.

https://www.ncbi.nlm.nih.gov/pubmed/23123794

Elderberry

A Review of the Antiviral Properties of Black Elder (Sambucus nigra L.) Products.

https://www.ncbi.nlm.nih.gov/pubmed/28198157

Randomized study of the efficacy and safety of oral elderberry extract in the treatment of influenza A and B virus infections.

https://www.ncbi.nlm.nih.gov/pubmed/15080016

Licorice

An Extract of Glycyrrhiza glabra (GutGard) Alleviates Symptoms of Functional Dyspepsia: A Randomized, Double-Blind, Placebo-Controlled Study

https://www.ncbi.nlm.nih.gov/pmc/articles/PMC3123991/

To evaluate of the effect of adding licorice to the standard treatment regimen of **Helicobacter pylori**

https://www.sciencedirect.com/science/article/pii/S141386
7016301696

Antiviral Activity of Glycyrrhizin against Hepatitis C
Virus *In Vitro*

https://www.ncbi.nlm.nih.gov/pmc/articles/PMC3715454/

Stress

Effects of stress on immune function: the good, the bad,
and the beautiful.

https://www.ncbi.nlm.nih.gov/pubmed/24798553

Sleep and Immune function

https://www.ncbi.nlm.nih.gov/pmc/articles/PMC3256323/

Emotional Wellbeing

How do our emotional affect immune response?

https://www.medicalnewstoday.com/articles/324090

APPENDIX II. CORONAVIRUS, COLD AND FLU SYMPTOMS

Symptoms	Coronavirus Symptoms range from mild to severe	Cold Gradual onset of symptoms	Flu Abrupt onset of symptoms
Fever	Common	Rare	Common
Fatigue	Sometimes	Sometimes	Common
Cough	Common* (usually dry)	Mild	Common* (usually dry)
Sneezing	No	Common	No
Aches and pains	Sometimes	Common	Common
Runny or stuffy nose	Rare	Common	Sometimes
Sore throat	Sometimes	Common	Sometimes
Diarrhea	Rare	No	Sometimes for children
Headaches	Sometimes	Rare	Common
Shortness of breath	Sometimes	No	No

Sources: World Health Organization, Centers for Disease Control and Prevention

I have been working on this book for more than a year, however, at the time of publishing this book, coronavirus pandemic has spread around the world and has caused great havoc in people's lives around the world. Even though this book about general information on the immune system and viruses, I thought readers may find the above table from the World Health Organization (WHO) above useful.